Thais de Brito Caldeira
Letícia Alves Teófilo

MENTAL HEALTH, SPIRITUALITY AND RELIGION

Thais de Brito Caldeira
Letícia Alves Teófilo

MENTAL HEALTH, SPIRITUALITY AND RELIGION

A REVIEW

ScienciaScripts

Imprint

Any brand names and product names mentioned in this book are subject to trademark, brand or patent protection and are trademarks or registered trademarks of their respective holders. The use of brand names, product names, common names, trade names, product descriptions etc. even without a particular marking in this work is in no way to be construed to mean that such names may be regarded as unrestricted in respect of trademark and brand protection legislation and could thus be used by anyone.

Cover image: www.ingimage.com

This book is a translation from the original published under ISBN 978-620-4-19247-5.

Publisher:
Sciencia Scripts
is a trademark of
Dodo Books Indian Ocean Ltd., member of the OmniScriptum S.R.L Publishing group
str. A.Russo 15, of. 61, Chisinau-2068, Republic of Moldova Europe
Printed at: see last page
ISBN: 978-620-4-04144-5

MENTAL HEALTH, SPIRITUALITY AND RELIGION:

A REVIEW

THAÍS DE BRITO CALDEIRA

LETICIA ALVES TEÓFILO

MONTES CLAROS - MG

2020

BIOGRAPHY OF THE AUTHORS

I am Thais de Brito Caldeira, from Minas Gerais, 27 years old. I started my medical degree in 2015. Medicine came to complete my being in all the biopsychosocial aspect. Being a doctor for me is synonymous with gift, of Divine trust and intense responsibility. Throughout the course I fell in love with Mental Health, because I understood and saw in practice the importance that the mind plays in the whole context of the health of any individual and, at the same time, awakened the will to help bring back the meaning of life for many who lost their lives while still alive. With this, I decided that this is the medical area to which I will dedicate myself with intense love and commitment.

My name is Letícia Alves Teófilo, from Minas Gerais, 28 years old. Medicine came into my life as a breath, a breeze, a caress in the soul. Understanding the human being in all its context involves a deep study of their physical and mental conditions, and from this, a wonderful world of discoveries opens up. Therefore, being a doctor is a privilege, and I am proud to have chosen this path.

AUTHOR'S DEDICATION

I, Thais de Brito Caldeira, dedicate this chapter to God, source of real love; to my grandfather Ivan Caldeira (*in memorian*), to my parents, Marilia and Hiram, who are essential pillars in everything I fight and achieve; to my children Ivan and Isis who are my greatest treasures and to my husband Luis who is always by my side. Every victory I achieve in my life has a little bit of each one of you.

I, Letícia Alves Teófilo, dedicate this chapter first to God, support of my existence; to my parents, Zuleide and Eder, for always being by my side; to my fiancé Leonel, for all the support; to my brother Victor for being my other half. Finally, I thank life for the luck of having so much and for all the lives that crossed mine.

PREFACE

This study aimed to verify the relationship between spirituality, religion and mental health. For this, a literature review was conducted between the years 2015 and November 2020, in the electronic database Latin American and Caribbean Center on Health Sciences Information (Bireme) using the descriptors in Portuguese and English: "Saúde mental", "Espiritualidade", "Religião", "Mental health", "Spirituality" and "Religion", from the *Boolean* operators "AND" and "OR".

The eligibility criteria were articles in Portuguese and English. Theses, duplicate articles and those diverging from the central theme were excluded. Twenty-five articles were selected and used for the review.

As a result, twenty-three articles showed that there is a positive impact when considering the religious and spiritual context in the complementary treatment of the mental health patient, carrier of some disorder such as depression, anxiety, impulsivity and chemical dependency, or even those susceptible: oncology patients, chronic renal patients undergoing hemodialysis and the elderly in dementia. Only two articles did not observe clinical relevance of the issue raised.

Therefore, it can be concluded from this study that there is a positive relationship between mental health, religion and spirituality for patients with mental disorders.

Conflict of Interest Declaration: Nothing to declare.

CONTENT

1 . INTRODUCTION

The relationship between mental health with religion and/or spirituality is a subject of growing interest in the social, behavioral and health sciences, since the religious or spiritual experience has been identified as a tool to help face the daily difficulties that mental disorders can trigger in the life of an individual. [1]

Many studies corroborate the affirmation that spirituality or religion can bring advantages to the mental health of individuals with mental disorders,[1-23] since it has been observed that patients with mental disorders that have greater involvement with religion or spirituality have an improvement in the psychological state with a consequent evolution in mental health. [5]

These factors may have a contributive role in saving lives,[6] since they can positively influence how someone sees and feels his/her own life and his/her current health status. [7]

Mental Health is considered as a state in which the person is able to keep in balance with himself and with the social relations he establishes, despite the daily adversities. However, when people live unbalanced in society, unable to convert their possibilities into reality, mental illness is characterized. [24]

Religion can be understood as an organized system that encompasses dogmas and certain practices interconnected with the sacred, based on faith in a superior being. Through these rituals, including prayer, religion may offer emotional support, comfort, life purposes, answers to doubts, and hope for life to individuals who find themselves within this context. [1] It may also serve as a vehicle through which the person would express his/her spirituality based on good values and allowing the search for reflections on the self and his/her existential relationships beyond the earthly world.

Thus, religion can represent an important tool with positive influence on the mental health of those who believe in it. The religious or spiritual dimension is part of the structure of much of the human population, and can influence the health and disease process of the individual, [9] offering the person, encouragement, help along the way, healing of doubts, hope and faith. [1]

Spirituality, on the other hand, can be considered to be a connection between the individual's consciousness with his or her deepest self, deities, and the outside world. [2]

And, as a philosophical tool that results in the production of behaviors that can bring considerable benefits to the individual as hope, love, and faith. [7] Thus, it may be a way for the individual to obtain new meanings in relation to his mishaps and, thus, reorganize his experiences. Even when the patient does not have any religion, spirituality appears as an important dimension, linked to significant existential issues. [3]

In 2015, the Executive Committee of the World Psychiatric Association accepted a statement for consideration of patients' spirituality, religious beliefs and practices and   their relationship to the diagnosis and treatment of psychiatric illness should be considered essential tools of clinical history, training and professional development. [1]

Holistic health care is already a reality in most health centers around the world. It is known the advantages that religion and spirituality can bring to the life of a large part of the population that has some form of mental disorder. It is increasingly important to consider these competences when providing health services to patients with mental disorders. [1]

In view of all this context, and from the premise that the patient should be considered holistically in the entire biopsychosocial context, it is important that the religion and spirituality of the individual with mental disorder be considered during the approach to his treatment, since in many cases these factors are part of the essence and identity of the patients. Therefore, a literature review is justified in order to verify the relationship between spirituality, religion, and mental health.

2. MATERIALS AND METHODS

The work was elaborated from the electronic data library *BVS/BIREME,* including the general population related to mental health, being susceptible or having some disorder.

The descriptors used in Portuguese were: *"saúde mental"*, *"espiritualidade" and "religião",* and the corresponding ones in English: *"mental health", "spirituality", "religion". All of them* should be present in the researched articles.

The following algorithm was used, with a result of 4948 papers: tw:((tw:(mental health)) OR (tw:(mental health)) AND (tw:(religion)) OR (tw:(religion)) AND (tw:(spirituality)) OR (tw:(spirituality))) AND (fulltext:("1") AND mj:("Religion" OR "Spirituality" OR "Mental Health") AND la:("en" OR "en")) AND (year_cluster:[2015 TO 2020]).

The eligibility criteria were articles found in the period from 2015 to 2020, written in Portuguese and English, which underwent a screening, as they should be in accordance with the guidelines of the *Preferred Reporting Items for Systematic Reviews and Metaanalysis* (PRISMA).

The selected articles had their title and abstract evaluated. Those that were not in accordance with the main theme were not used.

In the first screening, the texts of the platform that fit the exclusion criteria were discarded: Duplicate texts, case reports, letters, articles that did not include the aforementioned descriptors in the abstract, books, book chapters, dissertations, theses, papers that did not include the aforementioned descriptors as the main subject, and all that were nct appropriate to the theme of the study. The flowchart of the integrated search is shown below (Figure 1).

Soon after, 233 articles were selected for title reading, resulting in 40 papers. All of them were read in full, and thus 25 articles were selected to be part of the review (Table 2).

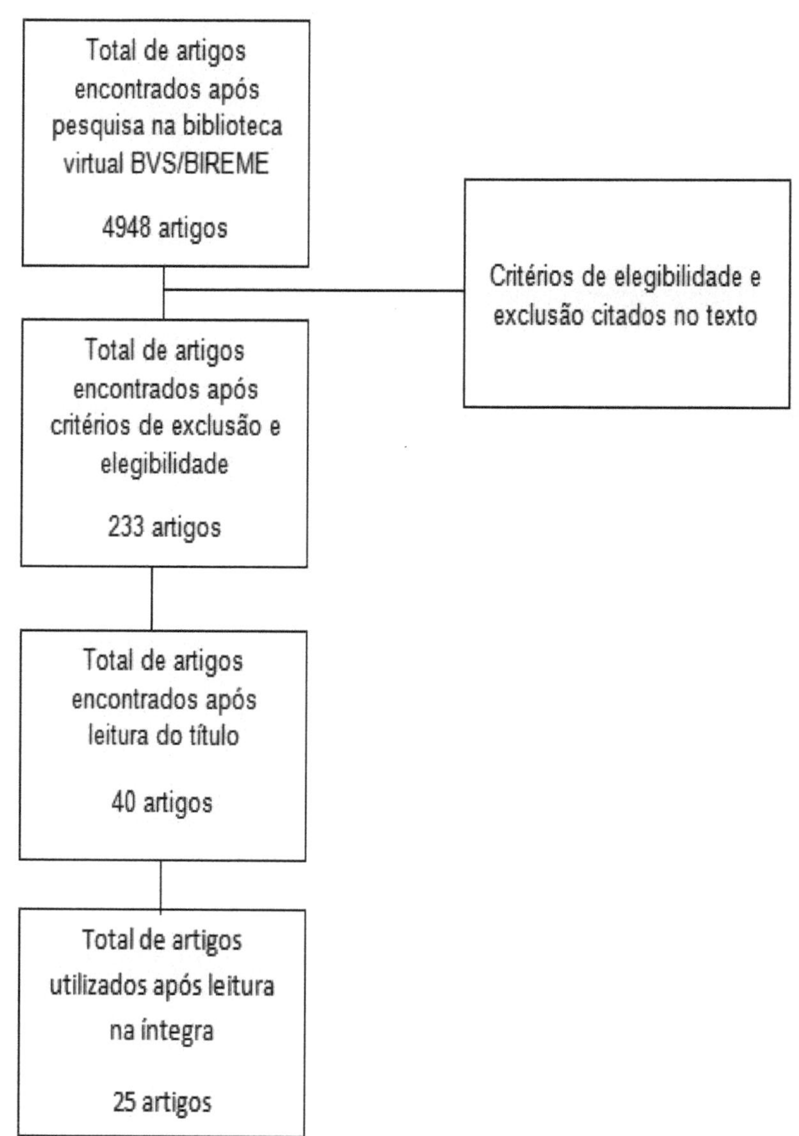

Figure 1- source own authorship.

Reference	Year	Author(s)	Title
1	2019	Figueredo et al.	Spirituality Directed to the Teaching of Nursing in Mental Health and Psychiatry Residency
2	2018	Lavorato et al.	The loose spirit: meanings of spirituality by nursing staff in psychiatry.
3	2015	Melo et al.	Correlation between religiosity, spirituality and quality of life: a literature review.
4	2015	André et a	Is religiosity a protective factor against suicidal behavior in bipolar I outpatients?
5	2016		Understanding spirituality

		Salimena et al.	for people with mental disorders: contributions to nursing care
6	2019	Ibrahim et al.	The role of social support and spiritual wellbeing in predicting suicidal ideation among marginalized adolescents in Malaysia.
7	2015	Souza et al. .	Spirituality, religiosity and personal beliefs of adolescents with cancer.
8	2015	Gonçalves et al	Religious and spiritual interventions in mental health care: a systematic review and meta-analysis of randomized controlled clinical trials.
9	2018	Loureiro et al.	The influence of spirituality and r

			religiousness on suicide risk and mental health of patients undergoing hemodialysis.
10	2017	Musa et al.	Spiritual Well-Being, Depression, and Stress Among Hemodialysis Patients in Jordan.
11	2019	Bovero et al.	The Spirituality in EndofLife Cancer Patients, in Relation to Anxiety, Depression, Coping Strategies and the Daily Spiritual Experiences: A CrossSectional Study.
12	2019	Baski and Sürücü et al.	Is spirituality an important variable as a predictor of emotional labor for nursing students?
13	2015	Bamonti et al	Spirituality attenuates the association between depression

			symptom severity and meaning in life.
14	2018	Sithey et al.	Socioeconomic, religious, spiritual and health factors associated with symptoms of common mental disorders: a crosssectional secondary analysis of data from Bhutan's Gross National Happiness Study
15	2015	Ribeiro and minayo et al.	Religious Therapeutic Communities in the recovery of drug addicts
16	2017	Zerbetto et al.	Religiosity and spirituality: mechanisms of positive influence on the life and treatment of alcoholics.

17	2016	Carneiro et al.	Religiosity/spirituality, mental health indicators and hematological parameters of nursing professionals.
18	2018	Paglione H.B et al	Quality of life, religiosity and anxious and depressive symptoms in liver transplant candidates
19	2019	Turke K.C. et al.	Depression, anxiety and spirituality in oncology patients.
20	2015	Vicente et al.	Religiosity, social support, and antidepressant use among the elderly: a population-based study
21	2017	Lac et al	Association between religious practice and risk of depression in older people in the subacute setting

22	2016	Nery et al.	Vulnerabilities, depression and religiosity in elderly patients admitted to an emergency unit
23	2018	Yoon et al.	symptoms in caregivers of patients with dementia.
24	2015	Lac et al.	Addressing Spiritual and Religious Inflences in Care Delivery.
25	2019	Alminhana et al.	Religious/spiritual experiences: healthy or pathological dissociation?

Figure 2- source own authorship.

3. RESULTS

After careful analysis, it was noticed that 23 articles consider that there is a positive impact when considering the religious and spiritual context in the complementary treatment of a patient in mental health, such as patients with depression, anxiety, impulsivity, chemical dependency, cancer patients, and the elderly, who are therefore susceptible to mental illness.

Only 02 articles were not favorable, and one of them believes there is no positive or negative influence when observing the aspects mentioned in the patient.

The benefits were broken down in table 3.

GROUP	RESULT
Cancer patients in palliative care	Source of strength, having lower intensity of depressive symptoms
Anxiety	Reduces symptoms
Marginalized adolescents and haemodialysis patients	Reduced suicidal thinking.
Bipolar Disorder	Reduced tendency to suicidal ideation and lower level of impulsivity
Mood, personality, or adjustment disorder	Fewer depressive symptoms and greater meaning in life

Alcohol dependent	Resilience, self-efficacy and hope in coping with alcohol dependence.
Nursing health professionals working in the outpatient units of the Clinical Hospital of the Federal University of the Triangulo Mineiro.	Less stress, depression, higher positive affect, and better immunity (based on WBC, neutrophil, and iga scores).
Patients candidates for liver transplantation and patients with cancer	Better quality of life, as they had fewer symptoms of anxiety and depression
Elderly	Less likely to use antidepressant medication

Figure 3- source own authorship.

4. DISCUSSION - MENTAL HEALTH, SPIRITUALITY AND RELIGION: A REVIEW

In most of the studies[1-23] researched, it was observed that spirituality or religion may exert a protective effect on mental health against the adversities imposed on the life of an individual with some mental disorder.

In contrast, in only two articles, no advantages were noted in the association between religion, spirituality and mental health. [25,26] As in one study that compared the presence of mental disorders in people with strong religious association with those with weak or absent religious connection and concluded that there was no significant difference between them. [26]

Another study reported that high levels of spirituality attenuate depressive symptoms, but that they are not very significant. [25]

A study conducted by Melo and collaborators in 2015,[3] found a positive correlation between religiosity/spirituality and coping with mental disorders. [23] Which is in line with the work of Salimena and collaborators,[5] who observed that greater intensities of religious and spiritual involvement are positively related to psychological well-being, such as contentment with life, happiness, positive affect and high morale, better physical and mental health.

Clinical trials that evaluated the effects of religious and spiritual intervention, showed benefits in comparison with control groups, such as reduction of clinical symptoms, especially of anxiety levels. [8]

These findings corroborate another study that found a considerable reduction in anxiety levels and a tendency to improve depression when considering the religious or spiritual context in approaches to patients with mental disorders. [7]

In another study[6] that addressed the role of social support and spiritual well-being among marginalized adolescents with suicidal ideation in Malaysia, it was found that highly religious youth are more optimistic and believe they can overcome life's obstacles, being less prone to suicidal behavior.

In the same sense, a research with 2nd, 3rd and 4th grade students attending the School of Health of a state university in southeastern Turkey reveals that nursing students with strong spirituality better manage their emotions during clinical practices. [12]

Another research, which was a cross-sectional study[4] including 164 patients with bipolar disorder type I, concluded that these patients who had religious affiliation had a lower tendency to suicidal ideation and a lower level of impulsiveness.

In another study[24] involving 55 adults who sought mental health outpatient clinics for treatment of mood, personality or adaptation disorders, the hypothesis that there is an association between severity of depressive symptoms and low spirituality with a consequent lower sense of meaning in life was supported.

In the same sense, a research conducted in Bhutan,[13] pointed out that increased spirituality and belief in a higher being are protective factors for common mental disorders.

Another study involving 53 nursing health professionals working in the Outpatient Units of the Hospital das Clinicas of the Universidade Federal do Triângulo Mineiro with great religious commitment, it was found that these professionals presented less stress and depression, as well as greater positive affect and better immunity. The dimension of organizational religiosity, which means the frequent participation of employees in religious meetings, is related to greater body immunity. The results of this study identified a relationship between religion and spirituality, mental health indicators and hematological parameters, demonstrating that the more religious and spiritualist nursing professionals present better mental health, greater immunity, based on the scores of leukocytes, neutrophils and *IgA*, in addition to better health perception. [16]

Paglione and other collaborators in 2019,[17] conducted a study involving patients who were candidates for liver transplantation, in which they found that the vast majority of these patients progressed with symptoms of anxiety disorder and depressive disorder. Foram encontrado dados que reforçam uma associação positiva da melhora da qualidade de vida desses pacientes com o envolvimento religioso. Os achados reforçam a necessidade de a equipe de saúde utilizar a religiosidade dos pacientes como uma estratégia de enfrentamento da doença.

Still in the aforementioned sense, a descriptive, cross-sectional and observational study [18] with cancer patients found that there was a positive relationship between low levels of anxiety and depression when the religious and spiritual context of these patients was considered and addressed. [15]

The daily spirit such as feeling touched by the beauty of creation or feeling the desire to be closer to or in union with God may represent a source of strength, for patients with terminal cancer who are at the end of life. In this context spiritual well-being becomes an important property in the palliative care of these patients, because daily spiritual experiences cause spiritual well-being in these patients and assist them for a better psychological health status. [11]

Having spiritual beliefs such as faith and greater meaning of life are associated with lower suicide risk and better mental health among patients who will need to undergo the hemodialysis process. [9]

Still in this context, a study[10] that included Jordanian Muslim patients on hemodialysis revealed that depression, anxiety and stress are common feelings in these patients and that, in addition, they usually suffer from spiritual and existential disorders.

The medium and high levels of religious well-being and religiosity, in this study, revealed that these dimensions are important for the lives of these people during the suffering of this process and the disease. A study covering patients with cancer and with a short life prognosis found that religious practice is useful in dealing with depression among these individuals. [11]

Regarding drug addicts, some churches evangelize in communities and recovery centers in order to complement drug therapy with religious treatment, based on a moral model that considers drug use as a distancing from God. The transforming capacity of faith is the most important element in this process. [14]

Considering the context of alcoholics dependents, a work carried out with these patients in treatment, it was concluded that those who participate in religious cult have more tranquility, personal comfort and more positive spiritual states. Alcohol users believe that the advantage of spirituality is in the progression of inner strength for health care and inner strengthening. These aspects intensify the capacity for resilience, self-efficacy, and hope in coping with alcohol dependence. The individual tries to replace the periods of increased consumption of alcohol by other activities, especially those related to religious practice, which aim to divert him from addiction. While religion enables reflections on self-care and identification of limits to conduct life, with prayer as a resource that promotes spiritual strengthening and belief in the hope that God can guide them in the best way to conduct their own lives, indicating better alternatives to overcome the problems faced. [15]

A research covering elderly people[19] who attended religious services more frequently, demonstrated that they were less likely to use antidepressant medications. In the same sense, a cross-sectional study[20] reported that religiosity was related to lower levels of depression in elderly people.

And, when considering caregivers of individuals with dementia, religiosity/spirituality can help to alleviate negative effects such as stress, which can be triggered in these caregivers. [21]

Holistic health care is a reality in some health centers around the world, however, when assessing the level of knowledge of health students on the subject that involves subjective dimensions such as spirituality and religiosity, a gap between techniques and care application is observed. It would be important to promote a dialogue between the pedagogical spheres and those of health care in order to think of proposals regarding implementation projects and public policies aimed at the care of the population susceptible to or bearing mental disorders. [1]

The findings provide some *insights* that both spirituality-religion and social support can greatly contribute to saving lives. [6] Given this context, it is important to explore and understand the benefits that the religious and/or spiritual dimension can bring to the individual with mental disorder, since these factors can help in the treatment and, consequenty, in the clinical improvement of the patient.

As a limitation of the study, the scarcity of studies addressing negative factors in the relationship between religion, spirituality and mental health can be reported.

5. CONCLUSION

Religion, spirituality and mental health is an important field that deserves to be increasingly studied and approached as complementary therapy in mental health, since it can be an important tool in the balance of the psychic functions of an individual. Therefore, it can indeed contribute to the mental health of a patient susceptible to or already suffering from a mental disorder. Furthermore, it is important that the practices related to the religious and spiritual context of the patient be encouraged by society, family, friends and health professionals, so that individuals may have more engagement and understand more about the importance of being inserted in this scenario. We believe that this study brings contributions to the health area, for with the course of research it was perceived that this relationship - religion, spirituality and mental health - deserves to be more incorporated and explored in clinical practices and in the curricula of health students. And finally, it is worth mentioning that we used a database of relevant data, encompassing the last 5 years, in order to obtain more updated data for this work.

6 . REFERENCES

1. Figueredo LP, Junior AC, Silva JCMC, Prates JG, Oliveira
   MAF. Spirituality Directed to the Teaching of Nursing
   Residency in Mental Health and Psychiatry. REVISA. 2019;
   8(3): 246-54. Doi:
   https://doi.org/10.36239/revisa.v8.n3.p246a254

2. Lavorato-Neto G, Rodrgues L, Turato ER, Campos CJG.
   The loose spirit: meanings of spirituality by nursing staff in
   psychiatry. Rev. Bras. Enferm. [Internet]. 2018 [cited 2020
   Nov 01];
   71(2): 280-88. Available at:
   http://www.scielo.br/scielo.php?script=sci_arttext&pid=S0034
   -71672018000200280&lng=pt.

3. Melo CF, Sampaio IS, Souza DLA, Pinto NS. Correlation
   between religiosity, spirituality and quality of life: a literature
   review. Estud. pesqui. psicol. [online]. 2015; 15(2): 447-64.
   ISSN 1808-4281.

4. Caribé AC, Studart P, Bezerra-Filho S, Brietzke E, Nunes Noto
   M, Vianna-Sulzbach M, *et al.* Is religiosity a protective factor
   against suicidal behavior in bipolar I outpatients? J Affect
   Disord. 2015; 1(186):156-61. doi: 10.1016/j.jad.2015.07.024.
   epub 2015 Jul 29. PMID: 26241664.

5. Salimena AMO, Ferrugini RRB, Melo MCSC, Amorim TV. Understanding spirituality for people with mental disorder: contributions to nursing care. Rev. Gaúcha Enferm. [Internet]. 2016 [cited 2020 Aug 11]; 37(3): e51934. Available from: http://www.scielo.br/scielo.php?script=sci_arttext&pid=S1983 -14472016000300401&lng=pt.　　　Epub　　25-Aug-2016. https://doi.org/10.1590/1983-1447.2016.03.51934.

6. Ibrahim N, Che Din N, Ahmad M, Amit N, Ghazali SE, Wahab S, Abdul Kadir NB, Halim FW, Halim MRT. The role of social support and spiritual wellbeing in predicting suicidal ideation among marginalized adolescents in Malaysia. BMC Public Health. 2019; 13;19(Suppl 4):553. doi: 10.1186/s12889-019-6861-7. PMID: 31196009; PMCID: PMC6565529.

7. Souza VM, Frizzo HCF, Paiva MHP, Bousso RS, Santos AS. Spirituality, religiosity and personal beliefs of adolescents with cancer. Rev. Bras. Enferm. [Internet]. 2015 [cited 2020 Nov 11];　　　68(5):　　　791-96.　　　Available　　　from: http://www.scielo.br/scielo.php?script=sci_arttext&pid=S0034 -71672015000500791&lng=en. https://doi.org/10.1590/0034-7167.2015680504i.

8. Gonçalves JP, Lucchetti G, Menezes PR, Vallada H. Religious and spiritual interventions in mental health care: a systematic review and meta-analysis of randomized controlled clinical trials.　　Psychol　　Med.　　2015;45(14):2937-49.　　doi: 10.1017/S0033291715001166. PMID: 26200715.

9. Loureiro ACT, Coelho MCR, Coutinho FB, Borges LH, Lucchetti G. The influence of spirituality and religiousness on suicide risk and mental health of patients undergoing hemodialysis. Compr. Psychiatry. 2018; 80: 39-45. https://doi.org/10.1016/j.comppsych.2017.08.004

10.Musa AS, Pevalin DJ, Al Khalaileh MAA. Spiritual Well-Being, Depression, and Stress Among Hemodialysis Patients in Jordan. J Holist Nurs. 2018;36(4):354-65. doi: 10.1177/0898980101117736686. Epub 2017 Nov 1. PMID: 29173010.

11.Bovero A, Tosi C, Botto R, Opezzo M, Giono-Calvetto F, Torta R. The Spirituality in End-of-Life Cancer Patients, in Relation to Anxiety, Depression, Coping Strategies and the Daily Spiritual Experiences: A Cross-Sectional Study. J Relig Health. 2019; 58(6):2144-60. doi: 10.1007/s10943-019-00849-z. PMID: 31165319.

12.Baski A, Sürücü HA. Is spirituality an important variable as the predictor of emotional labor for nursing students? Nurse Educ Today. 2019; 79:135-41. https://doi.org/10.1016/j.nedt.2019.05.025

13.Sithey G, Li M, Wen LM, Kelly PJ, Clarke K. Socioeconomic, religious, spiritual and health factors associated with symptoms of common mental disorders: a cross-sectional secondary analysis of data from Bhutan's Gross National

Happiness Study, 2015. BMJ Open 2018;8:e018202. doi:10.1136/bmjopen-2017-018202

14.Ribeiro FML, Minayo MCS. As Comunidades Terapêuticas religiosas na recuperação de dependentes de Drogas. Interface (Botucatu). 2015; 19(54):515-26. DOI: 10.1590/1807-57622014.0571

15.Zerbetto SR, Gonçalves AMS, Santile N, Galera SAF, Acorinte AC, Giovannetti G. Religiosity and spirituality: mechanisms of positive influence on the life and treatment of alcoholics. Esc. Anna Nery [Internet]. 2017 [cited September 05, 2020]; 21 (1): e20170005. Available from: http://www.scielo.br/scielo.php?script=sci_arttext&pid=S1414 81452017000100205&lng=en. https://doi.org/10.5935/1414-8145.20170005 .

16.Carneiro EM, Arantes JP, Silva DAAS, Catarino JS, Junior VR, Borges MF. Religiosity/spirituality, mental health indicators and hematological parameters of nursing professionals. Rev Enferm Assistência à saúde [Online]. 2020; 9(1):64-77. DOI: 10.18554 / reas.v9i1.3796.

17.Paglione HB, Oliveira PC, Mucci S, Roza BA, Schirmer J. Quality of life, religiosity, and anxiety and depressive symptoms in liver transplantation candidates. Rev Esc Enferm USP. 2019; 53:e03459. DOI: http://dx.doi.org/10.1590/S1980-220X2018010203459

18. Turke KC, Canonaco JS, Artioli T, Lima MSS, Batlle AR, Oliveira FCP et *al*. Depression, anxiety and spirituality in oncology patients. Rev. Assoc. Med. Bras. [Internet]. 2020 [cited 2020 Nov 11] ; 66(7): 960-65. Available from: http://www.scielo.br/scielo.php?script=sci_arttext&pid=S0104 42302020000700960&lng=en. https://doi.org/10.1590/1806-9282.66.7.960.

19. Vicente ART, Castro-Costa E, Firmo JOA, Lima-Costa MF, Filho AIL. Religiousness, social support and the use of antidepressants
among the elderly: a population-based study. Ciênc. saúde coletiva [Internet]. 2018 [cited November 06, 2020]; 23(3): 963-71. Disponível em: http://www.scielo.br/scielo.php?script=sci_arttext&pid=S1413 -81232018000300963&lng=en. https://doi.org/10.1590/1413-81232018233.05922016 .

20. Lac A, Austin N, Lemke R, S Poojary, Hunter P. Association between religious practice and risk of depression in older people in the subacute setting. AJA Inc. 2017; 36(2): E31 E34. https://doi.org/10.1111/ajag.12384

21. Yoon KH, Moon YS, Lee Y, Choi SH, Moon SY, Seo SW, *et al*. The moderating effect of religiosity on caregiving burden and depressive symptoms in caregivers of patients with dementia. Aging & Mental Health. 2016; 22(1):141-47. DOI: 10.1080 / 13607863.2016.1232366

22. LeDoux J, Mann C, Demoratz M, Young J. Addressing Spiritual and Religious Influences in Care Delivery. Prof Case Manag. 2019; 24(3):142-47. DOI: 10.1097/NCM.0000000000000346. PMID: 30946252. Alminhana LO, Menezes JA. Experiências religiosas/espirituais:

23. healthy or pathological dissociation? Horizonte, Belo Horizonte. 2016; 14(41):122-43. DOI -10.5752/P.2175-5841.2016v14n41p122

24. Waidman MAP, Jouclas VMG, Stefanelli MC. Family and mental illness. Fam Saúde Desenv. 1999;1(2):27-32.

25. Bamonti P, Lombardi S, Duberstein PR, King DA, Orden KAV. Spirituality attenuates the association between depression symptom severity and meaning in life. 2015; 20(5): 494-99. DOI: 10.1080 / 13607863.2015.1021752.http://dx.doi.org/10.1080/13607863.2015.1021752

26. Nery BLS, Cruz KCT, Faustino AM, Santos CTB. Vulnerabilities, depression and religiosity in elderly hospitalized in an emergency unit. Rev Gaúcha Enferm. 2018;39:e2017-0184. doi: https://doi.org/10.1590/1983-1447.2018.2017-0184.

Contributions

All authors participated in the conception and design of the study, analysis and interpretation of data, writing or relevant critical review of the intellectual content of the manuscript, final approval of the version to be published, and are responsible for all aspects of the work, including ensuring its accuracy and completeness.

Correspondence:

Thais de Brito Caldeira

Rua Desembargador Veloso, 1061, downtown

39390-000- Bocaiuva - MG

Telephone: +55 (38) 999173839

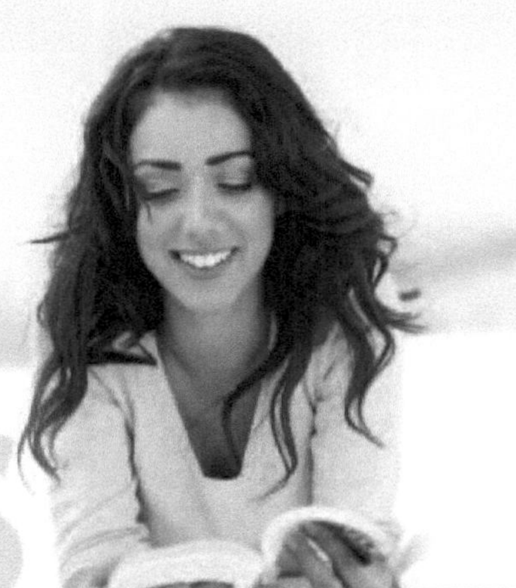

yes
I want morebooks!

Buy your books fast and straightforward online - at one of world's fastest growing online book stores! Environmentally sound due to Print-on-Demand technologies.

Buy your books online at
www.morebooks.shop

Kaufen Sie Ihre Bücher schnell und unkompliziert online – auf einer der am schnellsten wachsenden Buchhandelsplattformen weltweit! Dank Print-On-Demand umwelt- und ressourcenschonend produziert.

Bücher schneller online kaufen
www.morebooks.shop

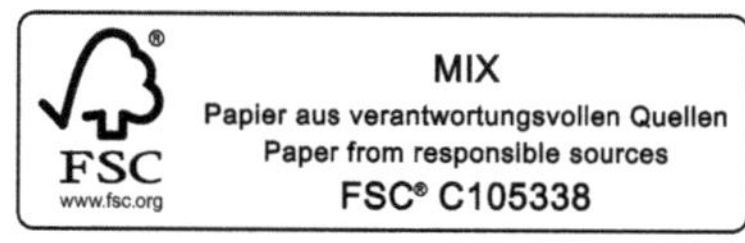

Printed by Books on Demand GmbH, Norderstedt / Germany